.wash

virginia mae nash

1

SPECIAL THANKS

TO KINDLE ALONGSIDE AMAZON WHO HAVE COLLABORATED TO ATTAIN

A SIGNATURE STYLE FOR PUBLISHED WORKS OF ALL SORTS.

<u>QUOTE</u>

my mother

"…you would not understand."

PRISCILLA ANN THOMPSON NASH, May 17,1924 – October 12, 2018

<u>QUOTE</u>

"Change the way you look at things, and things change the way they look."

DR. WAYNE W. DYER, author, _The Power of Intention_

JUNE, TWENTY-ONE, TWO-THOUSAND TWENTY

PRINTING OF MY SOLUTIONS IS INSTIGATED BY THE 2020, RUN OF COVID, A COMPLICATED GLOBAL DISCOMFORT. THESE RECIPES ASSIST EXPELATION OF THE LIFE CYCLES WITHIN US WHICH CAN CAUSE COMPLICATED DISCOMFORT.

1981, MY EXPOSURE TO VISUAL AND TACTILE INFORMATION POSITIONS MY UMBILICLE TO SEEK SOLUTION. PROMOTING MOTION WITH INSIGHT TO AN END HAS DRIVEN ME TO SEEK NOTHING BUT A COMFORTABLE SOLUTION. SOLUTION TO SIT IN TO PUT YOUR FEET IN TO RELAX IN. PRODUCTIVE BATHING SOLUTION TO RELEASE IN.

PARASITE ENTIMOLOGY WITHIN THE HUMAN HOST VARIES ABOUT THIRTY-EIGHT THOUSAND TIMES DUE TO SPECIES. PARASITES THAT   MISS   THE OPPORTUNITY TO EXPEL NATURALLY, STICK AROUND. THEY ARE   BLOCKED FROM RELEASE. OPPORTUNIST JOIN WITH THE BODY AND DERIGIBLE INTERNALLY WITH A TOPICAL APTITUDE.

FORTY-FIVE MINUTE BATHINGS ARE KEY TO FULL TOPICAL TISSUE HYDRATION.   A GOOD SOAK ALLOWS FOR HYDRO OSMOTIC PRESSURE TO BUILD AGAINST TISSUE OTHERWISE INACCESSIBLE.   THIS PRESSURE OFFERS OPPORTUNITY TO PROMOTE PARASITE MOTION AND THE POTENTIAL FOR ERADICATION FROM THE BODY. THE TOPICAL TISSUE IS A PIEACE OF ART, A MASTERPEICE TO WORK. SKIN IS THE LARGEST ORGAN AND THE LARGEST EXPELING ORGAN. SKIN TISSUE EMBODIES US AND WILL CONTINUE TOO.

EMBODY THE BATH   **GET CONDITIONED**   **GET WET**

MY NEW VOUGE

virginia mae nash

devoted to results - dedicated to solution

Dedication to my three children,

Priscilla, Hudson and

Magdelyn.

CAUTION/WARNING

ANY CONTRAINDICATION TO YOUR HEALTH SHOULD ONLY BE ADJUSTED BY YOUR PHYSICIAN

HOT WATER

ADJUST TO HEAT SLOWLY

UTILIZE PRODUCT WARNING

KEEP AWAY FROM EYES MOUTH

TABLE OF CONTENTS

in the bald

in the shower

condition

SLIPPAGE FACTOR – HIGH

NECESSITY

FOOT TUB

1 BOTTLE HAIR CONDITIONER

TOWEL FOR SHOWER FLOOR

INSTRUCTION

PRESOAK FEET FOR 45 MINUTES IN 1/2 BOTTLE OF CONDITIONER

APPLY 1/4 BOTTLE OF CONDITIONER TO CROWN ELBOWS KNEES NAILS WHILE SOAKING FEET

SHOWER IN WARM WATER WHILE <u>SLOWLY</u> APPLYING LAST 1/4 BOTTLE OF CONDITIONER TO CROWN

RINSE THOROUGHLY

paste

KEEP OUT OF EYES

NECESSITY

1 TUBE TOOTHPASTE

LIGHT WEIGHT LOOSE FITTING LONG SLEEVE SHIRT

LIGHT WEIGHT LOOSE FITTING PAJAMA PANT

INSTRUCTION

APPLY TOOTHPASTE TO CROWN HAIR LINE ELBOWS KNEES NAILS HIP BONES TAIL BONE <u>SPINE</u> FOOT PAD ANKLE BONES BEHIND EARS RIB CAGE SHIN

USE TILL TUBE IS EMPTY

DRESS

LEAVE ON 45 MINUTES

RINSE WELL IN WARM SHOWER

soap

NECESSITY

2 BARS SOAP

WASH CLOTH

INSTRUCTION

WRAP SOAP IN WASH CLOTH

SHOWER TILL ALL SOAP IS GONE

dry

NECESSITY

1 BAR SOAP

INSTRUCTION

RUB BAR SOAP OVER ENTIRE BODY

SHOWER OFF IN LUKEWARM WATER

charcoal

NECESSITY

8 CHARCOAL BRIQUETS

INSTRUCTION

RUB 1 BRIQUET AT A TIME ON BODY IN WARM SHOWER

not just anywhere

waxing

NECESSITY

BODY LOTION

THREAD WAX

INSTRUCTION

APPLY BODY LOTION

RUB WAX GENTLY ONTO CROWN HAIR LINE ELBOWS KNEES <u>NAILS</u> HIP BONES TAIL BONE SPINE FOOT PAD ANKLE BONES AROUND EARS RIB CAGE SHIN

repellent

NECESSITY

1 SPRAY BOTTLE BED BUG REPELLENT

INSTRUCTION

APPLY REPELLENT TO SCALP HAIR LINE EARS

ALLOW TO DRY

bleach dip

NECESSITY

1 SMALL BOTTLE BLEACH

SMALL BOWL

INSTRUCTION

POUR SOME BLEACH INTO SMALL BOWL

DIP NAILS IN BLEACH FOR 40 SECONDS

PAINT TOENAILS WITH BLEACH USING FINGERTIPS

ALLOW TO DRY

acetone dip

NECESSITY

1 BOTTLE CONDITIONED NAIL POLISH REMOVER

INSTRUCTION

APPLY TO CROWN ELBOWS KNEES AND NAILS

ALLOW TO DRY

REPEAT

foot tubbing

soda

NECESSITY

1 BOX BAKING SODA

LIQUID LAUNDRY DETERGENT

INSTRUCTION

POUR 1/2 BOX BAKING SODA INTO FOOT TUB

ADD 1/2 INCH LAUNDRY DETERGENT

SOAK FOOT PAD AND TOENAILS ONLY

SOAK 45 MINUTES OR LONGER

water

INSTRUCTION

FILL FOOT TUB WITH HOT WATER

GET IN CAUTIOUSLY ADJUSTING TOES FIRST

SOAK 45 MINUTES OR LONGER

coconut

SLIPPAGE FACTOR – HIGH

NECESSITY

COCONUT OIL

DURABLE SOCKS

INSTRUCTION

MEASURE 1 CUP COCONUT OIL INTO FOOT TUB

WORK OIL ON FEET WITH FEET

45 MINUTES OR LONGER

PUT ON SOCKS DIRECTLY OR WIPE OFF WITH TOWEL

flea/tick

NECESSITY

1 CAN FLEA/TICK SPRAY

TOWEL

INSTRUCTION

SPRAY 1 CAN FLEA/TICK SPRAY INTO FOOT TUB

FOOT PAD AND TOENAIL ONLY APPLICATION

45 MINUTES OR LONGER

WIPE OFF FOOT PAD WITH TOWEL

bed bug

NECESSITY

1 CAN BED BUG SPRAY

TOWEL

INSTRUCTION

SPRAY 1 CAN BED BUG SPRAY INTO FOOT TUB

FOOT PAD AND TOENAIL ONLY APPLICATION

45 MINUTES OR LONGER

WIPE OFF FOOT PAD WITH TOWEL

condition

NECESSITY

1 BOTTLE HAIR CONDITIONER

TOWEL

INSTRUCTION

MEASURE 1 1/2 CUPS HAIR CONDITIONER INTO FOOT TUB

WORK CONDITIONER ON FEET WITH FEET

45 MINUTES OR LONGER WIPE CONDITIONER OFF WITH TOWEL

sodium

NECESSITY

1 BOX ROCK SALT

INSTRUCTION

POUR 1 BOX ROCK SALT INTO FOOT TUB

FILL FOOT TUB WITH HOT WATER

GET IN CAUTIOUSLY ADJUSTING TOES FIRST

SOAK 45 MINUTES OR LONGER

salicylic

NECESSITY

1 BOTTLE BABY ASPRIN

INSTRUCTION

FILL FOOT TUB WITH HOT WATER

GET IN CAUTIOUSLY ADJUSTING TOES FIRST

ADD 20 BABY ASPRIN TO FOOT TUB

SOAK 45 MINUTES OR LONGER

soap

NECESSITY

1 BAR SOAP

WASH CLOTH

INSTRUCTION

FILL FOOT TUB WITH HOT WATER

GET IN CAUTIOUSLY ADJUSTING TOES FIRST

ADD BAR SOAP AND WASH CLOTH

WORK BAR SOAP AND WASH CLOTH ON FEET WITH FEET

ginger

NECESSITY

1 CHILLED QUART GINGER ALE

1 LIME FROZEN WHOLE

INSTRUCTION

POUR GINGER ALE INTO FOOT TUB

ADD WHOLE FROZEN LIME

SOAK 45 MINUTES OR LONGER

in the tub

bubble

NECESSITY

1 BIG BOTTLE BUBBLE BATH

INSTRUCTION

POUR 1 BIG BOTTLE BUBBLE BATH INTO TUB

FILL TUB WITH HOT WATER

GET IN CAUTIOUSLY ADJUSTING TOES FIRST

SOAK 45 MINUTES

jello

NECESSITY

1 LARGE BOX LIME OR LEMON JELLO

4 FABRIC SOFTENER SHEETS

INSTRUCTION

PUT JELLO AND FABRIC SHEETS INTO TUB

FILL TUB WITH HOT WATER

GET IN CAUTIOUSLY ADJUSTING TOES FIRST

SOAK 45 MINUTES

cold/flu

NECESSITY

4 MUG PACKS COLD/FLU REMEDY

INSTRUCTION

FILL TUB WITH HOT WATER

OPEN AND EMPTY INTO TUB 4 MUG PACKS COLD/FLU REMEDY

GET IN CAUTIOUSLY ADJUSTING TOES FIRST

SOAK 45 MINUTES OR LONGER

condition

NECESSITY

1 BOTTLE FABRIC CONDITIONER

4 FABRIC SOFTENER SHEETS

INSTRUCTION

POUR 2 CUPS FABRIC CONDITIONER IN TUB WHERE YOU WILL SIT

FILL TUB WITH HOT WATER

GET IN CAUTIOUSLY ADJUSTING TOES FIRST

USE FABRIC SHEETS AS WASH CLOTHS

SOAK 45 MINUTES

REHEAT AS NECESSARY

shaving cream

NECESSITY

1 CAN SHAVING CREAM

INSTRUCTION

APPLY SHAVING CREAM TO ENTIRE BODY

USE ENTIRE CAN

LEAVE ON TILL MOSTLY DRY

FILL TUB WITH HOT WATER

GET IN CAUTIOUSLY ADJUSTING TOES FIRST

SOAK 45 MINUTES OR LONGER

REHEAT AS NECESSARY

sunscreen

NECESSITY

1 BIG BOTTLE 35 OR HIGHER SUNSCREEN LOTION

INSTRUCTION

APPLY SUNSCREEN TO ENTIRE BODY

USE ENTIRE BOTTLE

LEAVE ON TILL MOSTLY DRY

FILL TUB WITH HOT WATER

GET IN CAUTIOUSLY ADJUSTING TOES FIRST

SOAK 45 MINUTES OR LONGER

REHEAT AS NECESSARY

Baby

EXTREMLY SLIPPERY

SLIPPAGE FACTOR – HIGH

NECESSITY

1 BOTTLE BABY OIL

3 WASH CLOTHS

SEVERAL TOWELS

BABY BATH BASIN

INSTRUCTION

PLACE WASH CLOTH IN BASIN

POUR 1/2 CUP BABY OIL ON TOWEL IN BASIN WHERE BABIES TAIL BONE AND BOTTOM WILL SIT

FILL BASIN WITH WARM WATER

LAY BABY ON WASH TOWEL GENTLY

GIVE BABY A 45 MINUTE SOAK

USE HANDS WITH TOWEL TO CONTROL SLIPPAGE

USE AS MANY TOWELS AS NECESSARY

KEEP ALERT TO BABY AND WATER TEMPERATURE

WARM WATER IF NECESSARY

mineral

SLIPPAGE FACTOR – HIGH

NECESSITY

1 BOTTLE MINERAL OIL

TUB TOWEL

INSTRUCTION

FILL TUB WITH HOT WATER

USE BATH TOWEL IN TUB TO SIT ON

POUR 1 BOTTLE MINERAL OIL ON BATH TOWEL IN TUB

GET IN CAUTIOUSLY ADJUSTING TOES FIRST

SIT ON OILED TOWEL

SOAK 45 MINUTES

AIR DRY

unbubble

NECESSITY

1 BIG BOTTLE BUBBLE BATH

INSTRUCTION

FILL TUB WITH HOT WATER

USE BATH TOWEL IN TUB TO SIT ON

POUR 1 BIG BOTTLE BUBBLE BATH ON BATH TOWEL IN TUB

GET IN CAUTIOUSLY ADJUSTING TOES FIRST

SIT ON BUBBLE BATH TOWEL

SOAK 45 MINUTES

body wax

NECESSITY

THREAD WAX

INSTRUCTION

FILL TUB WITH HOT WATER

GET IN CAUTIOUSLY ADJUSTING TOES FIRST, WORK THREAD WAX ONTO SKIN

MINIMUM 45 MINUTES

AIR DRY

coffee oil

SLIPPAGE FACTOR – HIGH

NECESSITY

1 BOTTLE MINERAL OIL

INSTANT COFFEE

TOWEL

INSTRUCTION

FILL TUB WITH HOT WATER

PLACE TOWEL ON FLOOR

ADD 2 CUPS DRY INSTANT COFFEE

GET IN CAUTIOUSLY ADJUSTING TOES FIRST

SOAK 45 MINUTES OR LONGER

REHEAT WATER IF NECESSARY

in the bald

paste smear

NECESSITY

1 TUBE TOOTHPASTE

INSTRUCTION

APPLY PASTE TO SCALP HAIR LINE EARS

LET SIT 2 HOURS

FRESH WATER RINSE

repellent

NECESSITY

1 SPRAY BOTTLE FLEA AND TICK REPELLENT

INSTRUCTION

APPLY TO SCALP HAIR LINE EARS

 LET DRY COMPLETELY

bald smear

NECESSITY

LEMON JUICE

LIME JUICE

COCONUT OIL

PLASTIC BAG TO COVER SCALP

DRY WASH CLOTH

INSTRUCTION

APPLY 4 DROPS LEMON JUICE TO CROWN

APPLY 4 DROPS LIME JUICE TO CROWN

SMEAR COCONUT OIL ON SCALP AND EARS EXTEND LIBERALLY PAST HAIRLINE

COVER SCALP AND EARS WITH PLASTIC

SECURE PLASTIC

LEAVE ON 12 HOURS

PULL PLASTIC

RUB-SCRUB HEAD WITH DRY WASH CLOTH

waxing

NECESSITY

THREAD WAX

LOTION

INSTRUCTION

APPLY LOTION TO HEAD

RUB WAX ON HEAD

DRYING THEN LAYERING IS ADVISED

caffeine slick

SLIPPAGE FACTOR – HIGH

NECESSITY

1 CHOCOLATE MINT

INSTANT COFFEE

COFFEE CUP

SKI HAT

INSTRUCTION

PUT CHOCOLATE MINT IN A COFFEE CUP

ADD TWO OUNCES HOT WATER

ADD 1 TABLESPOON INSTANT COFFEE

LET COOL

DIP FINGERS AND APPLY SLICK TO SCALP HAIR LINE EARS

PUT HAT ON TO COVER EARS AND HAIRLINE

LEAVE ON 45 MINUTES

FRESH WATER RINSE